Copyright (c)

All rights reserved. No part of this publication may be reproduced, distributed, or transmitted in any form or by any means, including photocopying, recording, or other electronic or mechanical methods, without the prior written permission of the publisher, except in the case of brief quotation embodied in critical reviews and certain other noncommercial uses permitted by copyright law.

Contents

Introduction

Welcome to "The Complete Kegel Exercise for Men". We're going to take a trip through the Kegel exercises to obtain a thorough comprehension of their creation and purpose. In 1948, Kegel exercises were first described by Arnold Kegel for pelvic floor muscle strengthening. This was intended to help women recover after giving birth, since then, the Kegel exercise has developed into an essential part of health routines for both men and women.

What is Kegel Exercise for Men?

Kegel exercises for Men are also called Pelvic floor training, which include repeatedly contracting, and releasing the muscles, which are the muscles that support the prostate in men, the bladder, and the rectum.

The Essential of Pelvic Floor Muscle:

A profound understanding of the pelvic floor is fundamental to Kegel exercise. The anatomy is clarified in this section and the purpose of provide a strong for the study of Kegel exercises. To maintain core strength and general well-being, the pelvic floor plays a crucial role in maintaining overall health and core strength by supporting organs and regulating fecal and urine continence.

Important of Kegel Exercises for Men:

Now that we have laid the basis by comprehending the history and structure of Kegel exercises, Lets discuss why these exercises are important for men.

Promoting Well-Being:

1. Core Strength: Kegel exercises improve general strength. Improving the power of the pelvic floor muscles has a beneficial effect on the body's basic strength, stability, and posture.

2. Controlling Pelvic Pain: A man's quality of life can be seriously affected by persistent pelvic pain. Understanding how Kegel exercises, work when executed appropriately,

helps reduce pelvic pain and the discomfort that goes along with it.

Sexual Health:

1. Erectile Function: Kegel exercises are essential for maintaining and enhancing erection. By keeping the muscles of the pelvic floor stronger, Men can have a beneficial effect on genital blood circulation, which can enhance erectile function.

2. Ejaculating control: One important component of sexual health is the capacity for control over ejaculation. This section covers how Kegel exercises give men the tools they need to better regulate their ejaculation. Strengthening the couple's sexual happiness.

3. Feelings and Libido: Strong pelvic floor muscles can improve desire and sex. Understand the complex relationship between Kegel exercises and increased libido, promote increased satisfied intimate life.

Cultivating Prostate Wellness:

1. Reducing Risk: For men, prostate health is an important concern, and Kegel exercises are a preventative method of lowering risk. Find out how using your pelvic floor muscles can help keep your prostate healthy and reduce the possibility of problems related to the prostate.

2. Supplemental Care: For anyone living with disorders related to the prostate, Kegel exercises can be a helpful supplement to medical care.

Determine the Pelvic Floor Muscles

We are going to set out on an organized expedition to learn the subtle skill of recognizing and disconnecting the false muscles of the pelvic floor. It is essential to have this fundamental ability for Kegel exercises to be effective. We follow a thorough manual that breaks the procedure down into doable parts and provides information on typical traps to guarantee accurate muscle activation.

Comprehending the Landscape of the Pelvic Floor:

Before taking any concrete action, understanding the complexities of pelvic floor anatomy is essential. This comprises the tendons, muscles, and connective tissues that support this important area's basis. Equipped with this understanding, the procedure for identifying and the process of identifying the pelvic floor muscles becomes more knowledgeable and intuitive.

A Comprehensive Guide to Identification:

1. Relaxation Preparation: Look for a pleasant, quiet environment. Choose a comfortable position, such as sitting or lying down, to aid in concentrating and a calm atmosphere that helps with muscle identification.

2. Mental Illusion: Develop a mental picture of the pelvic floor muscles in your mind. Imagine

the area between the pubic bone and the tailbone, reaching the perineum, which refers to the area in men between the scrotum and the anus.

3. Interrupting Urination Technique: Try to stop the flow temporarily when urinating. The pelvic floor muscles are the ones triggering this disruption. Nevertheless, It is not recommended to use this technique frequently when urinating.

4. Anal Tightness: Imagine drawing your anus higher, as though trying to stop the gas from passing through. The pelvic floor muscles are used in this process. Remain calm in your thighs, and buttocks, and belly when performing this exercise.

Common Mistakes to Avoid:

1. Abdominal Contraction Excessive: Watch out for inadvertently activating the abdominal muscles rather than releasing the pelvic floor. Put your surroundings' comfort first for accuracy.

2. Holding Your Breath: during your muscles, try not to hold your breath as this can cause tension. Throughout the procedure, keep your breathing regular and comfortable.

In this section, we discuss the important steps to take to properly prepare before performing Kegel exercises. Making sure your Kegel exercise is fun and successful requires preparation. Establishing a favorable atmosphere and embracing the appropriate perspective, to get the most out of these revolutionary pelvic floor exercises, we walk you through the preliminary phase.

Setting a Friendly Environment:

1. Select a Quiet Area: choose a peaceful and comfortable area where you won't be interrupted and can concentrate. This provides a setting that is beneficial for unwinding and focusing.

2. Relaxing Clothes: Put on a casual and comfortable dress that permits free movement. This guarantees that you will complete Kegel exercises without difficulty or interference.

Warm-Up Exercises:

1. Pelvic Shifts: To warm up the pelvic floor muscles, gently move your pelvis. This includes, whether lying down or seated, shifting the pelvis forward and backward.

2. Inhaling deeply: Breathe deeply and diaphragmatically. This causes the body to relax and foster calmness, make sure you begin kegel exercises with a calm and concentrated attitude.

Get Materials:

1. Biofeedback Tools: If preferred, think about implementing biofeedback tools to get immediate feedback on your muscles' activation. These materials can assist you to improve your technique and have a better knowledge of the exercises.

2. Incorporate Resistance: As you improve, you could decide to use resistance instruments, For instance, weighted Kegel balls. They enhance the scope of things you do and help you develop stronger pelvic floor muscles.

In this section, we look into the foundation of the basic Kegal exercise, intended to improve the tone and strength of the pelvic floor muscles. Whether Kegels are new to you or looking forward to know more technique, this section will help you establish a solid foundation for pelvic health.

1. Determine Your Initial Position:

Either lie down on your back or take a comfortable chair. Retain a neutral posture with a straight spine. This prepares your pelvic floor muscles for active use.

2. Identify Your Pelvic Floor Muscles:

Take the actions listed in Determine the Pelvic Floor Muscles (Chapter 2 of this book) to help find and isolate your pelvic floor muscles. Try to stop the flow temporarily when urinating. The pelvic floor muscles are the ones triggering this disruption.

3. Lift and Tense:

Imagine pulling these muscles up, away from the chair or floor. The core of a Kegel exercise is this deliberate contraction. Take a deep breath in then when you release the breath, tense the muscles in your pelvic floor.

4. Hold and calm:

Hold the contraction for three to five seconds, making sure your breathing remains stable

Let go of the tightness and Give your pelvic floor muscles the same amount of time to fully calm. The foundation of every repetition is this rhythmic pattern.

5. Continue the Cycle:

Execute a series of ten rounds, deliberately tensing and relaxing your pelvic floor muscles. As the exercises grow more comfortable for you, increase the rounds.

6. The Key To Success Is Consistency:

Include this series of basic Kegel exercises in your workout routine three times a day at the minimum. Set a routine that fits in with your everyday activities.

7. Improve Gradually:

So as your pelvic floor gets stronger, attempt to use longer contractions, continuing for ten seconds at most. Furthermore, examine whether you can increase the total number of repeats in every set.

8. Track Your Progress:

To track your progress, keep a journal. Keep records of any changes that occur to your muscle control. Acknowledge accomplishments and use the notebook to evaluate yourself.

Including Kegel in Everyday Activities

By incorporating Kegel exercise into your everyday routine, you can fully realize their potential. This useful book provides doable strategies and pointers to help you incorporate Kegel exercises into your daily routine in an easy and fulfilling way that promotes pelvic health and enhances your general well-being.

1. Morning Wake-Up Routine:

As part of your daily routine, begin your day with a series of Kegel exercises. Kegel exercises can help you feel good about the hours ahead, whether you're getting ready for the day or just resting in bed.

2. Breaks from Desk Work:

Kegel exercises can be incorporated into your workday by scheduling brief pauses for pelvic floor exercises. Perform discrete sets of Kegel exercises to maintain muscle activation and break up extended periods of sitting, whether at a desk or in a virtual meeting.

3. Kegels and Posture Check:

Kegel exercises should be combined with healthy posture habits. Engage your pelvic floor muscles whenever you check and correct your posture, whether you're standing, walking, or even just sitting at a computer. This dual emphasis improves pelvic health as well as spinal alignment.

4. Every Day Reminders:

Throughout the day, utilize sticky notes or digital reminders on your phone to remind yourself to perform Kegel exercises. Regular reminders help to form a habit loop that makes it simpler to remember and incorporate Kegel exercises into your daily routine.

5. Bathroom Kegel Exercises:

Connect Kegel exercises to rest periods. Once your main task is over, stop for a series of Kegel exercises. This practice helps improve bladder control in addition to strengthening the habit.

6. Exercise Combo:

Include Kegel exercises in your normal workout regimen. Workout with Kegel exercises whether you're running, doing yoga, or working out at the gym. This combination increases total muscle activation and makes a workout regimen more all-encompassing.

7. Evening Relaxation Routine:

Include Kegel exercises in your bedtime routine for relaxation. Whether you do Kegels at night as part of your stretching regimen, during meditation, or just before bed, it helps to maintain general pelvic health and muscular relaxation.

8. Kegel in pairs:

Turn Kegel exercises into a joint activity that you both do. Think about training with a partner, making it a fun pastime that improves closeness and communication.

Discover the benefits of Kegel exercises as an all-natural method of treating erectile dysfunction. This describes the relationship between erectile function and pelvic floor wellness, discussing successful techniques to incorporate Kegel exercises into your routine for enhanced sexual well-being.

1. Discovering the Connection between Erectile Function and Kegel Exercises

1. Improving Pelvic Blood Flow Strength:

Kegel exercises improve urinary blood circulation and long-lasting erections. Improving the pelvic floor muscles helps to enhance the vascular function necessary for erectile health.

2. Boosting Muscular Tone:

Frequent Kegel exercises boost tone, which is essential for maintaining erectile function. Better control over erections is facilitated by stronger muscles.

3. Improving Perceptual Awareness:

Kegel promotes a mind body connection. The overall quality of sexual experiences and arousal may benefit from this heightened sensitivity.

2. The Kegel Exercise for Erectile Dysfunction Management

1. Basic Kegel Exercises:

Start with the basic Kegel exercises described in Chapter 4 of this book. Before moving on to more specialized techniques, you must grasp the fundamentals.

2. Progressive Contractions:

Increase the span and force of contractions gradually. Ascend to longer holds, aiming for up to 10 seconds, starting with shorter contractions. Over time, the pelvic floor muscles become stronger.

3. Including Opposition:

Consider more complex methods by using opposition equipment like Kegel balls these pieces of equipment give your exercise routine an additional level of complexity and increase the pelvic floor muscles' involvement.

3. Strategies for Addressing Erectile Dysfunction(ED)

1. Reverse Kegel:

Adding reverse Kegel exercises to enhance standard contractions. By deliberately tensing and relaxing the pelvic floor muscles, these exercises enhance general muscle balance and flexibility.

2. Integration of Breath work:

Combine Kegel exercises with deep breathing through the diaphragm. This synchrony makes it easier to relax and encourages the best possible blood flow to the pelvic area, which supports the health of the erection.

4. Lifestyle Factors for the Best Outcomes

1. Cardiovascular Workout:

Include cardiovascular workouts in your daily or weekly schedule. Walking, running, and cycling are exercises that improve cardiovascular health, favorably affecting the body's blood flow throughout, including the urinary area.

2. Eating Balanced Diet:

Eat a diet high in nutrients and well-balanced. Antioxidants, vitamins, and mineral-rich foods promote vascular health and enhance general well-being, which includes erectile performance.

5. Improving Ejaculatory Control

A weaker pelvic floor could make delaying ejaculation more difficult. Kegel exercises aid in making these muscles stronger.

To start:

1. Locate the appropriate muscles: To locate your muscles on the pelvic floor, cease urinating in midstream. Alternatively, tense the muscles preventing you from passing gas.

Your pelvic floor muscles are used in both actions.

2. Barbell Hip Thrust: This will increase your gluten strength, hip range of motion, and thrust capability. Place your feet flat on the floor in front of you and place your upper back on a bench. Lift your hips till your body forms a straight line from your shoulders to your knees while supporting a barbell on your hip crease. After a count, hold, and then carefully move back to the beginning position.

3. Compound Workout: Your body's largest muscles are the focus of this workout.

Maintain a shoulder-width distance between your feet while supporting a barbell across your upper chest. You have two options: either extends your wrists to support the weight on your fingers, or cross your arms to support the weight. Be careful not to hunch your back, lower your body till your thighs are parallel to the floor by pushing your hips back and bending your knees. Press your heels into the ground to propel yourself back up to the starting position with force.

4. Squat Jumps: Squat Jumps increase blood supply to the pelvic area, increasing the intensity of orgasms. Stand with your feet shoulder-width apart. Bend your knees and sit back with your hips to begin the exercise. Go as low as you can before launching yourself skyward. Throughout the exercise, maintain a straight back and an upturned head.Try to

land gently to lessen the force on your knees,
and then lower yourself before repeating.

What is Prostate and its function?

In men, the prostate is a little gland that sits under the bladder. It encircles the urethra, and its role is to generate seminal fluid, which is an essential part of semen.

The Benefits of kegel Exercises on Prostate Wellness:

1. It Helps Building Up the Pelvic Floor Muscles:

Kegel exercises focus on the muscles of the pelvic floor, which are essential for maintaining the prostate. Kegel exercises that strengthen these muscles improve the general health of the prostate.

2. Better Blood Circulation:

Kegel exercises improve blood flow to the prostate and surrounding pelvic area. Better blood flow supports proper performance and contributes to preventing problems such as prostatitis.

3. Preventing Prostate Issues:

Kegel exercises can help avoid common prostate problems, by improving muscle tone and flexibility. Improved pelvic floor muscle control can have a beneficial effect on sexual and urinary function.

Kegel Exercises for Prostate Wellness:

1. Basic Kegel Exercises:

Start with the Kegel basics discussed in Chapter 4 of this book. Gaining proficiency in these basic motions paves the way for specific advantages in prostate health.

Progressive Contractions:

Increase the length and force of your Kegel exercises gradually. As you advance via these activities, their muscular power increases and the prostate is fully supported.

3. Methods of Relaxation:

Include relaxing methods in your daily practice. Following each contraction, the pelvic floor muscles should be quickly and completely relaxed to increase flexibility and support a healthy prostate.

Advanced Kegel exercises entail harder methods to bolster and regulate the pelvic floor muscles even more. It is important to establish a strong foundation in fundamental Kegel exercises before undertaking advanced activities. Seek advice from a medical expert if you have any ailments or worries.

1. Isometric Contractions with Variation:

 i. Changing Contractions: Pelvic floor muscles in the front and rear should alternately be engaged and held while the other is released.
ii. Gradual Pulls: From mild to maximal, gradually raise the contraction's intensity, and then release it gradually.

2. Kegel Exercises That Are Dynamic

 i. Tilts of the Pelvis: Lift and lower the pelvis while using the pelvic floor muscles by combining Kegel contractions with pelvic tilts.

ii. Leg raises: It will test your balance and muscle coordination to lift one leg at a time while keeping a firm pelvic floor contraction.

3. Resistance Exercise

 i. Using resistance bands for Kegels: Use resistance bands to increase the external resistance, making the pelvic floor muscles work harder as they contract.

ii. Kegel exercises with weights: Gradually increase the load on the exercises by adding resistance with a tiny, safe weight (such as a weighted kegel ball).

4. Squeezing Balloons

i. A tiny, deflated balloon should be inserted into the rectum.

ii. Use the pelvic floor muscles to inflate the balloon as you perform Kegel contractions.

iii. To prevent overinflating, concentrate on precision and control.

5. Contractions in Elevators

i. Think of the muscles in your pelvic floor as a multi-story elevator.

ii. As you ascend, contract your muscles little by little, as though you were pausing at each floor, and then relax them gradually as you descend.

6. Coordinated Breathing

i. Align Kegel contractions with deep diaphragmatic breathing.

ii. Pelvic floor muscles tense as you breath, then relax.

7. Advanced Methods of Biofeedback

i. To monitor and improve contractions of the pelvic floor muscles, use biofeedback devices.

ii. Concentrate on reaching particular strength objectives and improving control.

8. Integration of Function

i. Use Kegel exercises in practical contexts, such as weightlifting or athletics.

ii. For practical strength, emphasize using your muscles in functional actions.

9. Mind-Body Link

i. Use visualization and mindfulness exercises to increase your awareness of the activation of your pelvic floor muscles.

ii. During Kegel exercises, link your physical control and mental focus.

10. Exercises with a Partner

 i. Investigate workouts that combine resistance and support with a partner for shared advantages.

 ii. In order to conduct partner-assisted exercises effectively, communication and understanding are essential.

Conclusion

"The Complete Kegel Exercise for Men" is a thorough manual that allows men to take charge of their general well-being and pelvic health. All through this manual, we have looked at the important of Kegel exercises for developing stronger pelvic muscles, and increased sexual function.

As we progressed through the many exercises and methods, it became clear that doing Kegel exercises regularly has a significant positive impact. From increased satisfaction during sexual activity to averting frequent health problems, like erectile dysfunction and urine incontinence, regular Kegel exercise has a significant impact.

Furthermore, the significance of mindfulness and appropriate methods in attaining the best outcomes has been underscored in this manual. By integrating clear instructions, and practical recommendations, we hoped to demystify the process and make it accessible for men of all ages.

In addition to embracing the activities in this guide, we hope that readers will develop a holistic perspective on their health. Understanding the connection between mental and physical health, achieving pelvic fitness becomes the first step in living a more satisfying and balanced life.

As you begin your Kegel exercise, keep in mind that consistency is essential. This book is an invitation to set out on a journey of self-discovery, empowerment, and better health, more than just a manual. May your dedication to pelvic wellness serve as the cornerstone for a more contented, self-assured, and healthy you.

www.ingramcontent.com/pod-product-compliance
Lightning Source LLC
Chambersburg PA
CBHW060815260726

48660CB00002B/962